# A Guide to Geocaching Fitness and Natural Nutrition

# Table of Contents

# Chapter 1. Introduction

Discover the joy of exploration coupled with the thrill of fitness with our exclusive Special Report: A Guide to Geocaching Fitness and Natural Nutrition! This comprehensive guide is tailor-made for you who yearn for adventure and also cherish the commitment to wellness. Whether you're a seasoned geocacher or just starting off on this fascinating journey, this guide is packed with vital information, tips, and advice that connect geocaching activities with physical fitness and natural nutrition. It's an inspiring combination of the joy of treasure hunting, the benefits of outdoor exercise, and the goodness of wholesome, natural foods. Buy this special report today and step out for an exciting venture towards a healthier you! Journey with us beyond the beaten tracks into nature's gym and kitchen, where the treasures don't just sparkle, they improve your life too!

# Chapter 2. The Wonders of Geocaching: A Comprehensive Introduction

Geocaching is a global, high-tech treasure hunt that merges the thrill of exploration with the wonders of technology. Participants employ GPS-enabled devices to hunt for hidden containers, known as "geocaches," while using coordinates that are posted online. But geocaching goes far beyond mere coordinates and containers—it's about adventure, discovery, and making unforgettable memories.

## 2.1. Understanding Geocaching

Before delving further into geocaching, it's essential to grasp a familiar understanding of what it entails. Geocaching is an outdoor recreational activity where people use coordinates and GPS devices to find hidden items, known as geocaches.

These geocaches vary in size, shape, and difficulty level. They may be as small as a fingertip or as large as a box, hidden anywhere from the heart of a city to the far-reaching ends of a hiking trail. Inside the geocache is a logbook for finders to sign and date, acknowledging their successful discovery. Sometimes, geocaches include trinkets or toys, allowing for a fun exchange—take an item and leave an item.

## 2.2. The History of Geocaching

The origin of geocaching dates back to May 3, 2000, coinciding with the "Great Blue Switch" event where the U.S. Government improved the Global Positioning System (GPS) significantly. The first-ever geocache was placed the following day by Dave Ulmer in Oregon, USA, containing a logbook, pencil, and various trinkets, igniting the tradition of item exchanges. Today, with more than 3 million geocaches around the world, it's a phenomenon enjoyed by individuals and families globally.

## 2.3. Equipment for Geocaching

The most basic equipment required for geocaching is a GPS device or a GPS-enabled smartphone. These are used to navigate to the coordinates specified on the geocache listing.

In addition to a GPS, here are other useful items: * Notebook and pen: To jot down notes or hints that might help in the search. * Tweezers: Useful for extracting logbooks from small geocaches. * Flashlight: Handy if the geocache is in a dark place or if you're geocaching at night. * Swag for trade: Small, inexpensive items to exchange. * Extra batteries or a portable charger: To ensure your GPS or smartphone stays powered throughout the adventure.

## 2.4. Rules of Geocaching

To maintain the spirit, fun, and fairness of the game, several unwritten rules have been established. These are guidelines for optimising the experience, both for the seekers and the hiders: 1. If you take something from the geocache, leave something of equal or greater value. 2. Write about your find in the cache logbook. 3. Log your experience online on the geocaching platform.

## 2.5. The Different Types of Geocaches

There are a variety of geocaches to discover. Here are some of the most common types: 1. Traditional Cache: The original type of geocache, it includes at least a container and a logbook. 2. Multi-cache: Involves multiple locations, with the final location being a physical container with a logbook inside. 3. Mystery or Puzzle Caches: These caches involve a puzzle that must be solved to determine the coordinates. 4. EarthCache: An EarthCache site educates individuals about a geological feature or aspect.

## 2.6. Geocaching and Community

Geocaching isn't just about the hunt; it's a highly social activity too. Enthusiasts often engage in gatherings known as 'geocaching events' hosted by fellow geocachers, which can range from basic meet-and-greets to large, organized festivals. These events are an excellent opportunity for newcomers to learn from the veterans and for seasoned players to share stories and experiences.

## 2.7. Geocaching and Fitness

Geocaching has a significant fitness aspect that often flies under the radar. Participants might find themselves walking, hiking, or even climbing during the pursuit of a cache. While it may not seem like it amidst the excitement of the hunt, every step taken is a step toward better physical health.

So whether it's the wish to explore your surroundings, the thrill of the hunt, the joy of discovering new things, or the satisfaction of physical exercise, geocaching has something for everyone. It carries a world of adventure waiting for you to uncover. And with each geocache, you write a page of your own colorful exploring story! Geocaching isn't a hobby; it's a journey of discovery, adventure, and fun. Let the geocaching adventure begin!

# Chapter 3. Geocaching 101: Equipment and Techniques

The thrills of geocaching come hand in hand with the need for the right gear and the correct techniques. As fascinating as the activity is, the success of your venture largely depends on your preparation. A well-assembled geocaching kit coupled with proper strategies can turn your expedition into an engaging and rewarding experience.

## 3.1. Getting Equipped: The Geocaching Kit

Planning your geocache quest begins with the assemblage of a well-stocked geocaching kit. There are some essentials, without which your experience might be rather incomplete or challenging. Here's a rundown:

*1+ | GPS or Smartphone with Geocaching App:*

The primary tool for a geocacher, a GPS device or a smartphone with a geocaching application will lead you to the geocaches. While GPS devices tend to be more accurate and resistant to environmental conditions, smartphones are convenient and multi-functional. Geocaching apps also usually include maps, logs, clue decryption tools, and user community features. There are many free and paid geocaching applications available.

*2+ | Compass:*

A handy tool to add a touch of traditional navigation to your modern geocaching experience. A compass can serve as a backup in areas with poor network coverage.

*3+ | Notebook & Pen:*

To jot down notes or clues you may stumble upon during your hunt. Also, many geocaches require or at least encourage you to sign a physical logbook inside the cache.

*4+ | Swag for Trading:*

It's customary, though not obligatory, to bring small trinkets for trade when you find a geocache. The rule of thumb: if you take something, leave something of equal or greater value.

*5+ | Flashlight:*

For those unexpected evening hunts or hidden caches in dark spaces, a flashlight can be incredibly valuable.

*6+ | Tweezers or Pick-up Tool:*

Some caches (especially small or micro ones) are too tight for human fingers. A small tool can help you extract the logbook or swag without damaging it.

*7+ | Spare Batteries/Power Bank:*

If your device runs out of charge in the middle of your adventure, you'll be thankful for that power backup.

*8+ | First Aid Kit:*

Safety first! Slips, scrapes, and scratches can happen. Be prepared to treat minor ailments with a basic kit.

*9+ | Water & Snacks:*

Hydrate and refuel yourself with water and energy-dense foods like nuts or energy bars to keep the fun going.

# 3.2. Mastering the Techniques: Geocaching Strategies

Armed with your geocaching kit, you're ready to step into the world of geocaching. However, a full geocaching kit won't be much help if you don't have the right approach to deciphering the geocaching clues and finding those caches. Here are some of the victories garnished techniques in the geocaching realm.

*1+ | Understanding the Coordinates:*

Geocaching is all about navigation, and it starts with the comprehension of coordinates - latitude and longitude to pinpoint a location down to a few meters. Be familiar not only with how to read coordinates but also with inputting the format that your GPS device or geocaching app requires.

*2+ | Decoding Geocaching Clues:*

Sometimes, finding a geocache needs a bit more than just coordinates. As a geocacher, you may have to decipher coded clues. Your geocaching app may host clue decrypters, or you can find them online.

*3+ | Observing Geo-senses:*

Over time, seasoned geocachers develop what is known as 'geo-senses'. This is the ability to spot potential cache hiding places or 'unnatural' things in the environment around where the cache should be located.

*4+ | Stealth:*

Remember, not everyone is aware of geocaching. The game relies on 'muggles' (non-geocachers) not interfering with the caches. When searching or placing a geocache, try to be discreet.

*5+ | Preserve Nature:*

Part of the appeal of geocaching is exploring the great outdoors. Always strive to leave no trace. If you move anything to access a cache, return it to its original position. The goal is to minimize the impact on the environment while maximizing the joy of the hunt!

*6+ | Log Your Find:*

Logging your find is critical. It's respectful communication to the cache owner and other hunters who may be after the same cache. With smartphone apps, you can log your find in real time at the location.

*7+ | Celebrate Your Finds!*

A central part of geocaching is the camaraderie. Don't forget to share your finds and experiences with your geocaching pals or through online platforms. They'll love to hear about your adventure!

Venture into a comprehensive blend of adventure, intellectual stimulation, physical exercise, and natural exploration with geocaching. Harness the excitement of the search, appreciate the joy of discovery, benefit from the greatness of being active, and ultimately connect closer with the environment, yourself, and your fellow geocachers. As you step into this whimsical world armed with your kit and these techniques, remember, it's not just about the find; the journey itself is the treasure; geocaching is all about creating unforgettable experiences and healthful memories. Happy Hunting!

# Chapter 4. Boosting Physical Activity Through Geocaching

Geocaching, often touted as the game played across the world by adventure seekers equipped with GPS devices, is not just an exciting pursuit but also a surprising boost to physical fitness. This adventure provides an opportunity to combine exercise with exploration in a unique and stimulating format. Geocaching prompts you to work out, without it feeling as arduous as traditional exercise often can. This chapter delves into how this exciting game can help you boost physical activity.

## 4.1. The Mechanics of Geocaching

The mechanics of geocaching are simple but infinitely variable, making it an accessible and adaptable exercise tool. To geocache, you use a GPS device to locate containers called 'geocaches' or 'caches' that are hidden in various locations all over the world. These containers could be anywhere – in your local park, on a city street, at the beach, or atop a mountain. The important aspect is that they are outdoors and getting to them almost always involves some degree of physical activity.

Geocaching often involves walking, climbing, trekking, or even swimming, with the intensity varying depending on the location of the cache. As a result, geocaching can offer moderate to high-intensity cardiovascular exercise, improving heart health, reducing the risk of cardiovascular diseases, and aiding in weight management.

## 4.2. Walking Towards Wellness

Walking is the most common physical activity associated with geocaching. On a typical cache hunt, you might find yourself walking slowly, intently examining your surroundings, or hiking at a brisk pace to reach the cache before anyone else. All these activities count towards your daily physical activity requirements.

According to the World Health Organization, adults should engage in at least 150 minutes of moderate-intensity, or 75 minutes of vigorous-intensity aerobic physical activity throughout the week. With geocaching, you'll likely exceed these recommended amounts without even realising it. The beauty lies in the unpredictability of the journey rather than the destination.

## 4.3. Intensifying Fitness Regime

Not all geocaches are a simple walk in the park. Many require climbing, mountain biking, cross country skiing, and other adventurous activities to get to. The challenge and adrenaline rush add an extra layer of motivation, turning a simple game into an enraptured quest that pushes you physically.

It's not just the cardiovascular system that benefits either; the strenuous activities associated with geocaching can improve skeletal muscle strength and endurance, respiratory capability, metabolic efficiency, bone density, and overall flexibility and balance.

## 4.4. Incidental Fitness and Mindfulness

One fascinating aspect of the geocaching-fitness connection is the incidental nature of the exercise. The focus of the activity is on the hunt, and the physical activity is almost inconspicuous. You are not walking or climbing because you have to, but because you want to find the cache. This perspective can make geocaching a very sustainable form of physical activity, because it takes the 'work' out of 'workout'.

Geocaching also encourages a form of mindfulness, where you are not just physically active, but mentally engrossed too. This conscious combination of mind and body contributes to overall well-being, and studies show that it can lead to better mental health and improved cognitive functioning.

# 4.5. Community and Social Interaction

Geocaching often involves teamwork and social interaction, which can be beneficial for both psychological wellbeing and increased physical activity. Group cache hunts encourage community engagement, stimulate friendly competition, and provide the motivation needed to push yourself further.

These social interactions can also provide increased safety, especially when attempting to locate caches in hard-to-reach areas or when introducing new physical activities such as rock-climbing or rafting.

In conclusion, geocaching can be an extremely beneficial method of boosting physical fitness. It wraps the aspects of a workout in a blanket of adventure, thereby serving the benefits of exercise whilst encouraging exploration and discovery. It's not just the treasure that's located at the end of the quest, but also a healthier version of you. Start your cache hunt today and uncover a world of wonders that promise wellness and more.

# Chapter 5. Interactive Fitness Regimes for Geocachers

Geocaching is more than just an adventure-come-treasure hunt, it is a catalyst for a plethora of fitness regimes, encouraging interactive physical activities while catering to the curiosity of the explorer within us.

## 5.1. Understanding the Geocaching Workout

Geocaching can be classified as a moderately intense physical activity, which involves plenty of walking, bending, lifting, and climbing—depending on the terrain and difficulty level of the cache. It keeps the heart rate elevated and works out different muscle groups, thereby helping in enhancing cardiovascular fitness, improving balance, agility and muscular strength.

Engaging in geocaching activities of varying intensity and duration, contributes to your weekly quota of physical activity. Depending on the difficulty, terrain, and distance of the geocaching expedition, it can satisfy low to moderate or even high-intensity workout requirements.

## 5.2. Incorporating Warm-ups and Cool-downs

As with any physical activity, each geocaching expedition should ideally begin with a warm-up session and end with a cool-down period. Warm-ups prepare your body for the workout ahead and minimize the risk of injury. Cool downs, on the other hand, help your body gradually transition from a state of vigorous activity to a rest state, preventing post-exercise issues like dizziness or fainting, and assisting in faster recovery.

**Warm Up**: Begin with a light walk or jog to get your heart rate up gradually. Follow this up with mobility exercises like arm swings, shoulder rolls, ankle rotations, and hip circles.

**Cool Down**: After completing the cache hunt, slow down your pace gradually before coming to a complete halt. Once your heart rate has slowed down, stretch out the muscles that you have used during the hunt.

# 5.3. Exploring Different Terrains for Varied Workouts

Different terrains challenge your body in different ways, providing varied workout experiences. When planning your geocaching adventure, consider exploring diverse landscapes for a mixed bag of physical challenges:

**Flat Terrains**: Ideal for beginners, flat terrains provide for a low-impact, cardiovascular workout. They are excellent for building endurance, lower body strength, and enhancing aerobic fitness.

**Hilly Terrains**: If you're looking to challenge yourself more, choose hilly terrains that demand more from you and contribute to an intensive cardiovascular workout. Climbing uphill helps develop leg strength, balance, and flexibility.

**Rugged Terrains**: For seasoned geocachers looking for a high-intensity workout, rugged terrains are the ideal choice. Navigating through rocky landscapes, crossing streams, and traversing trails in wooded areas can engage multiple muscle groups, leading to a comprehensive, full-body workout.

# 5.4. Combining Strength Training and Geocaching

For an optimized geocaching workout, incorporating strength training principles into your geocaching expedition can pay great dividends.

Resistance Band: Carry a light resistance band that can fit into your geocaching bag. While searching for your cache, take short breaks to perform a few resistance exercises such as squats, lunges, or band pull-aparts.

Body Weight Exercises: Utilize rest time or waiting periods to perform bodyweight exercises like push-ups, triceps dips or step-ups on logs, rocks or park benches.

# 5.5. Engaging in Group/Team Geocaching

Geocaching can be a fun group activity, enabling teamwork and further enhancing the concept of interactive fitness regimes. Group geocaching encourages friendly competition, leading to increased physical activity.

# 5.6. Periodically Monitoring Your Fitness Level

Track your resting heart rate, walking/running speed, or time taken to recover post-activity as an index of your fitness. Over time, with consistent geocaching activities, you'll observe a tangible improvement in these parameters.

# 5.7. Creating a Personalized Geocaching Fitness Regime

Finally, remember that the most effective fitness regime is one that is personalized. Start with your current fitness level, and then select the complexity and frequency of geocaching adventures accordingly. Carefully increasing the challenge over time can stimulate continuous adaptation and improvement, keeping your fitness journey both engaging and effective.

Embrace the adventurous spirit of geocaching, and use it as a tool to enhance physical fitness. Let the promise of discovery guide you to wellness, amid nature's charm and thrill. Happy Geocaching!

# Chapter 6. Decoding Nature: The Power of Outdoor Workouts

Exposing oneself to nature, breathing in the fresh air, feeling the warmth of the sunlight or the coolness of the breeze, can be both empowering and invigorating. Outdoor workouts not only provide an opportunity to engage with natural settings, but also exhibit a multitude of health benefits. They make fitness routines more enjoyable and fresh, and render them sustainable over an extended period.

## 6.1. Why Outdoor Workouts?

Outdoor workouts encompass a broad spectrum of physical activities and exercises conducted in open spaces, notably in natural environments. The great outdoors essentially acts as a natural gymnasium, providing an easily accessible, open-ended, and cost-free space for working out.

Outdoor workouts offer critical physical benefits. Working out in the open air can increase energy levels, boost mood, reduce fatigue, and lower blood pressure. This type of exercise is also associated with improved mental health, including eased symptoms of depression and anxiety.

Perhaps the most significant health benefit of outdoor workouts is the increased level of Vitamin D obtained through sunlight exposure. Vitamin D is crucial for maintaining strong bones, boosting the immune system, reducing inflammation, and facilitating the process of cellular regeneration.

# 6.2. The Power of Outdoor Workouts

Outdoor workouts have a two-fold power: they improve physical health and mental wellbeing. The physical benefits include enhanced cardiovascular health, increased muscle strength, flexibility and coordination, improved balance, and improved weight management.

Mental health perks of outdoor workouts are also notable. The process of exercising in a natural environment has been linked to improved mood, increased self-esteem, reduced stress, and enhanced cognitive function. A 2010 study published in the Journal 'Environmental Science & Technology' even suggested that as little as five minutes of exercise in a green space can significantly improve mood and self-esteem.

# 6.3. The Science behind Outdoor Workouts

When delving into the science of outdoor activities, multiple aspects come into play. Firstly, being in an outdoor setting can take us away from the everyday stressors. The natural light, the sounds of nature, and a change from our usual environments all play a part in promoting mental wellbeing.

When we exercise outdoors, our bodies release endorphins, the mood-elevating hormones. Further, the exposure to sunlight enables our bodies to synthesize vitamin D, which boosts our mood and bolsters our immune system.

Outdoor environments can often demand more from our bodies than indoor workouts. Walking or running on uneven terrain means the body has to adjust continuously and makes more significant demands on the system as compared to doing the same on a flat, man-made surface.

# 6.4. Geocaching Fitness: A New Perspective on Outdoor Workouts

Geocaching, the outdoor recreational activity of hunting for hidden items using GPS coordinates, perfectly combines the thrill of a treasure hunt and the benefits of outdoor workouts. It brings a novel perspective on fitness, synthesizing the physical health benefits and mental wellness aspects of outdoor workouts.

Finding caches involves a substantial amount of walking, digging, climbing, and even sprinting, all of which are excellent forms of physical activity. It brings the fun into fitness, making it less of a chore and more of a fun pursuit, thus ensuring that people are more committed to it and hence more likely to achieve their fitness goals.

It's hard to beat the thrill of locating a hidden cache. In the process, the geocacher experiences several physiological and psychological benefits. The cardiovascular system gets a boost with all the hikes and trails involved in hunting. Meditative aspects of being at one with nature can be as potent as mindfulness techniques for lowering stress and overall mental wellbeing.

In conclusion, the power of outdoor workouts lies in their dual ability to enhance physical health and support mental wellbeing. They offer an escape from the typical fitness routine and a chance to connect with the natural world, making workouts something to look forward to rather than a daunting task to complete. Specifically, adventure-based activities like geocaching amplify these benefits and mark an exciting turn in the realm of outdoor fitness. Geocaching fulfills the desire to explore and discover, resulting in an effective, enriching, and enjoyable fitness experience.

Exercise has always been fundamental to health and wellness. When coupled with the excitement of exploration and the vastness of nature, it propels your fitness journey to new horizons – reaping benefits for mind, body, and soul at once. So, step out, start your geocaching adventure and explore the power of outdoor workouts for yourself. It's time to decode nature. It's time to start living more healthily – and more adventurously.

# Chapter 7. A Beginner's Guide to Natural Nutrition

The concept of "Natural Nutrition" can seem overwhelming at first glance, but with the right guidance, it's an invigorating and healthy path to venture on. Whether fueling for long treks or finding the best refreshments in nature, understanding natural nutrition could not only spell success for your geocaching adventures but also a healthier lifestyle.

## 7.1. Understanding Natural Nutrition

Natural nutrition emphasizes consuming foods in their most organic and wholesome form - unprocessed and untreated. The aim is to fuel the body with nutrients that come unaltered from Mother Nature, providing maximal health benefits and limiting exposure to processed foods that could potentially harm the body with trans fats, artificial ingredients, and excessive sugars.

Let's first take a look at the macronutrients, which form the basis of natural nutrition: proteins, carbohydrates, and fats.

1. Proteins: Proteins are the building blocks of life. They're crucial for muscle development and repair, vital for those geocaching adventures that might test your physical limits.

2. Carbohydrates: Carbohydrates, especially complex ones, are our body's preferred source of energy. They provide the necessary fuel for those long hikes and strenuous digging.

3. Fats: While fats often get a bad reputation, healthy fats are vital for various body processes, including hormone production, nutrient absorption, and brain functions.

# 7.2. Essential Nutrient-Rich Foods

A few foods outshine the rest when it comes to the sheer powerhouse of nutrients they offer. Incorporating these into your diet can boost your health and ensure that you're energized for your geocaching adventures.

1. Leafy Greens: Leafy green vegetables such as spinach, kale and Swiss chard are packed with nutrition. They're a good source of fiber, vitamins A, C, K and several B-vitamins along with minerals like calcium, iron, potassium and magnesium.

2. Berries: Berries, particularly blueberries, raspberries and blackberries are rich in fiber, vitamins and potent antioxidants that can strengthen your immune system.

3. Legumes: Legumes such as beans, lentils, and peas are an excellent source of protein and fiber and are also enriched with vitamins and minerals.

4. Nuts and Seeds: Nuts such as almonds, walnuts, and seeds like flaxseeds, chia seeds are great sources of healthy fats, proteins, and fibers.

5. Whole Grains: Whole grains like quinoa, brown rice, and oatmeal contain more fiber and nutrients than their refined counterparts.

# 7.3. Planning your Natural Nutrition Diet

To implement natural nutrition, make a balanced diet plan using the food groups mentioned above. Aim for a variety of foods to cover all nutrients required by your body. Use each food group as a building block.

1. Meal Ideas: A smoothie for breakfast with leafy greens, chia seeds, mixed with fruits and a dollop of almond butter can be a

great start to the day. You could opt for a mixed legume-high protein salad for lunch, and perhaps a lean-protein like fish paired with quinoa and stir-fry vegetables for dinner.

2. Hydrating: Hydrating properly during geocaching is paramount. Don't rely solely on water, especially during longer geocaching hunts. Rehydration salts or fruit-infused water can help keep electrolyte balance.

3. Snacking: Healthy, nutrient-dense snacks like nuts and dried fruits or protein bars with minimal added sugars can provide sustained energy and satiety.

# 7.4. Barriers and Solutions to Natural Nutrition

While embracing natural nutrition, you may face challenges like sourcing natural and organic produce or resisting processed foods.

Sourcing Organic and Natural Food: It can be challenging to find organic food in your local grocery store, and when found, it may be expensive. Buying seasonally, shopping at farmer's markets or local farm shops, or even starting your own garden are productive ways to deal with this.

Resisting Processed Foods: It's hard not to give in to convenient, ready-to-eat foods. The key is to be prepared. Meal prep at the start of the week to ensure you have healthy options readily available.

Embracing natural nutrition isn't just about adjusting your diet—it's about adopting a lifestyle that values food for its ability to nourish, rebuild, and sustain us in our ventures, whether that involves geocaching or rebuilding one's health. By choosing foods closer to their natural state, you're investing in your body's well-being and your continued ability to discover and explore.

Remember, it's a journey, and any small step towards a natural and nourishing diet will ripple into a healthier and energized self ready to take on the next geocaching adventure.

# Chapter 8. Essential Foods for the Active Geocacher

The world of geocaching is one that's dominated by physical activity and the great outdoors. If you're an active geocacher or planning to join the ranks, it's vital that you fuel your body with the right nutrients to keep you energized, healthy, and ready to seek out those hidden containers. This section is dedicated to outlining the essential foods that every geocacher should consider incorporating into their diet.

## 8.1. Foods That Provide Energy

The energy to search for caches comes from the food you eat. Carbohydrates, proteins, and fats are the three macronutrients that provide energy and should be a staple part of your diet.

Whole grains like oats, brown rice, and quinoa are excellent sources of carbohydrates. They provide sustained energy and contain fiber, which is beneficial for digestion. Whole grain bread sandwiches with healthy fillings can make great meals before you head out geocaching.

For proteins, lean meats such as chicken and turkey are ideal choices. Vegan alternatives entail tofu, lentils or chickpeas, all of which are packed with protein. Proteins are essential for muscular health which is key when physically active.

Fats have been vilified in the past but they are crucial for energy and absorption of fat-soluble vitamins. Nuts, seeds, avocados, olive oil, and fatty fish are healthy fat sources.

# 8.2. Snacks for Sustained Stamina

Snacks are a vital component of a geocacher's nutrition plan. They help maintain blood sugar levels and provide much-needed energy on long expeditions. Here are some options:

- Trail Mix: A combination of nuts, seeds, dried fruits, and dark chocolate, can provide quick energy and maintain stamina.

- Fresh Fruits: Apples, bananas, and oranges are easy to carry and provide a good boost of natural sugars, fiber, and essential vitamins.

# 8.3. Hydration

Being outdoors, particularly in the heat, can quickly lead to dehydration. Carrying a water bottle is a must. You can also pack hydration tablets or opt for natural coconut water, which provides electrolytes and minerals lost during sweat.

# 8.4. Recovery Meals Post-Geocaching

Recovery meals are crucial in replenishing lost energy reserves and repairing worn-out muscles. After a geocaching adventure, your meal should have:

- Proteins: To repair muscle tissue. Choose from lean meats, tofu, eggs, or Greek yogurt.

- Carbohydrates: To replenish energy reserves. Prefer whole grains, sweet potatoes, or fruits.

- Fats: Particularly omega-3 fatty acids that have anti-inflammatory properties to speed up recovery.

# 8.5. Nutrient-Dense Foods

Fruits and vegetables are packed with vitamins, minerals, and antioxidants that support the immune system, enhance cellular repair, and combat oxidative stress caused by physical exertion.

- Berries: Rich in antioxidants and vitamins.

- Leafy greens: They offer an array of vitamins, fiber, and even some protein.

- Beetroot: Known for its capacity to enhance blood flow leading to improved physical performance.

# 8.6. Supplements

Though most nutrients can be received from a well-balanced diet, some individuals may benefit from supplements:

- Protein Powder: Useful for those not meeting their protein needs via food.

- Multivitamins: Provide a wide array of vitamins and minerals.

- Omega-3 capsules: Beneficial for those who don't regularly consume fatty fish.

Remember, nutrition is personal. What works for one geocacher might not work for another. Listen to your body and fuel it in a way that makes you feel good both inside and out. A well-fed geocacher is a successful one, so give yourself the advantage by fueling right!

# Chapter 9. Creating Nutrient-Rich Meals for Your Geocaching Journey

The connection between great nutrition and geocaching success can't be overstressed. To embark on a successful geocaching trip requires maintaining energy levels and staying sharp, which is primarily determined by the type of foods you consume. In this section, we're going to explore innovative recipes and meal ideas, focusing on nutrient-rich foods to fuel your journey.

## 9.1. Understanding Macros Before You Pack

To start with, it's essential to understand macronutrients: fats, proteins, and carbohydrates. They are the most vital because they provide energy in the form of calories.

Protein is a great source of extended energy, aids in muscle repair, and helps keep you full longer. Fish, poultry, lean meats, eggs, and plant proteins (like beans and lentils) are ideal.

Carbohydrates, especially complex ones from whole grains and vegetables, provide quick energy release. Fiber-rich carbs can assist in digestion and give a sustained release of energy, which is important for long excursions.

Although fats have been given a bad reputation, healthy fats are crucial for energy storage and insulation. Foods like avocados, nuts, seeds, and oils filled with omega-3 fatty acids can help reduce joint inflammation caused by extended physical exertion.

Do remember, though, balance is key. A healthy regime involves a mix of these macronutrients, rather than an excess of one.

# 9.2. Developing a Pre-geocaching Menu

Before a geocaching adventure, it's vital to energize your body with a balanced mix of protein, carbohydrates, and healthy fats.

Here's an easy and nutritious breakfast recipe to fuel up for a full day:

Recipe: Quinoa Porridge

| Ingredient | Quantity | Method |
| --- | --- | --- |
| Quinoa | 1 cup | Wash the quinoa thoroughly, then cook it in 2 cups of water till it's fluffy and the water is absorbed. |
| Almond milk | 1 cup | After the quinoa is cooked, add almond milk and stir until it heats up. |
| Mixed berries, fresh or frozen | 1 cup | Throw in the berries and simmer for another 2-3 minutes. You can add honey or a bit of pure maple syrup for natural sweetness. |
| Nuts and seeds mix (almonds, flaxseeds, pumpkin seeds) | 1/4 cup | Consider lightly toasting them for added crunch, then sprinkle over the porridge. |

This protein and fiber-rich breakfast will ensure a consistent energy release throughout your day.

# 9.3. Packable Nutrient-Dense Snacks

During geocaching, frequent snack breaks become necessary, especially if you're traversing challenging terrains. The aim is to have portable, non-perishable, and lightweight snacks providing quick energy.

Here are some ideas: - Homemade trail mix: Combine raw almonds, walnuts, sunflower seeds, pumpkin seeds, dried cherries, dark chocolate chips. - Banana or apple with a small packet of almond butter. - Whole grain wraps with almond butter, fresh fruits, and seeds. - A mix of fresh fruits (apples, oranges, berries) in a reusable container.

# 9.4. Staying Hydrated

Fluid intake is as essential as nutrient intake. Long outings, especially under the sun, can lead to dehydration. Carry adequate water, adding electrolyte tablets to a portion of it for replenishing any lost salts. Coconut water is another great natural alternative for hydration and electrolyte replenishment.

# 9.5. Post-geocaching Meal

Post-geocaching, it's time to restock lost nutrient stores and aid in muscle recovery. A balanced meal within an hour can prevent prolonged fatigue and muscle soreness.

Try this balanced dinner recipe:

Recipe: Grilled Chicken and Vegetable Bowl

| Ingredient | Quantity | Method |
| --- | --- | --- |
| Boneless chicken breast | 1 piece | Marinate chicken with lemon juice, garlic, olive oil, salt, and pepper. Grill until fully cooked. |
| Quinoa | 1 cup | Cook according to package instructions or use leftover quinoa from breakfast. |
| Assorted vegetables (bell pepper, broccoli, zucchini) | 2 cups | Chop the veggies and roast or grill them until they are just tender. |
| Dressing: Greek yogurt, lemon juice, garlic, dill, salt and pepper | To taste | Mix all ingredients together and pour over your bowl before eating. |

This hearty meal replenishes lost nutrients, repairs muscles, and fuels future adventures.

Remember, proper nutrition significantly affects your geocaching success. By taking care of dietary needs, you're ensuring a stronger, more enjoyable, and ultimately, successful venture. Nutrition and geocaching go hand-in-hand; each fuels the other in a cycle of wellness and adventure.

# Chapter 10. Aligning Geocaching Goals with Health Objectives

The intersection of adventure and wellness begins when your geocaching goals align seamlessly with your health objectives. The very nature of geocaching - hiking through varied terrains, analyzing clues, and hunting for hidden treasures - provides ample opportunities to boost physical fitness.

## 10.1. The Adventurous Path to Fitness

Geocaching isn't just about finding hidden treasures. Each trek to unearth a geocache offers a chance to enhance your physical wellbeing. Strapped with your GPS device and a rucksack brimming with essentials, you embark on a wild adventure that is more than a mere jog or run through a paved park. Every geocache hunt engages your legs in a hike, your core in navigating uneven terrains, and your arms in climbing or reaching out for the geocache.

For instance, an afternoon of geocaching can easily replace a typical gym session with added benefits. Instead of the treadmill, you have the open trails. Instead of the controlled climate of an enclosed gym, you have the natural elements playing with your endurance. And instead of being confined and surrounded by gym equipment, your senses are treated to the sights, sounds, and smells of nature that positively impact your overall wellbeing.

# 10.2. Integrating Goals

But like any fitness regimen, your geocaching ambitions should align with health objectives to ensure your activities are beneficial to your overall health.

Set realistic goals both for geocaching and your health. If your fitness level currently permits you to walk for 2 kilometers continuously, aim for caches that fall in this radius. As your endurance improves, expand your range to challenge yourself and boost physical conditioning further. However, it's essential to remember not to overextend yourself in your excitement to lay hands on difficult geocaches.

# 10.3. The Role of Natural Nutrition

Geocaching is energy-intensive, considering the terrain and the mental focus it demands. And just as the city park and the gym scale differently on the fitness levels due to the open-ended, challenging nature of the former, the food we consume also scales on a similar spectrum.

Natural nutrition — like geocaching — means going back to baser roots. Avoiding overly processed foods and embracing a diet full of a variety of whole foods such as fruits, vegetables, lean meats, and whole grains can provide the energy needed for your geocaching adventures and promote quicker recovery post-hikes.

Consider food as fuel. For a sport as physically demanding as geocaching, replenishing the calories burnt with nutrient-rich meals becomes significant. Incorporate complex carbohydrates, lean proteins, and healthy fats for balanced energy delivery throughout your geocaching journey.

# 10.4. Seeking Professional Guidance

If you're new to the world of geocaching or endeavoring to overhaul your lifestyle radically, reaching out to professionals like fitness coaches, registered dietitians, or medical practitioners can be immensely beneficial.

Fitness coaches can provide appropriate advice on physical training and exercises based on your current fitness levels to prepare you for the strenuous aspects of geocaching. Registered dietitians can help devise natural nutritional plans aligning with the increased physical activity geocaching brings.

When you align geocaching with health objectives, the hidden treasures are no longer just the caches you unearth, but also the increased stamina, improved cardiovascular health, enhanced muscular strength, and a holistic sense of well-being. Embark on your geocaching journey, step by step, cache by cache, towards your health goals.

# Chapter 11. Geocaching and Natural Nutrition: Charting Success Stories

From the verdant trails of Washington State to the mountains of Colorado, the geocaching community is filled with tales of changed lives and reclaimed health. These experiences, naturally woven with the threads of nutrition and adventures, paint the growing landscape of geocaching fitness. We have combed through endless narratives to bring you the most impactful stories—those charting the remarkable intersection of natural nutrition and geocaching.

## 11.1. A New Leaf: Martha's Story

Martha was stuck in a rut. Her zest for life was dwindling, her health was declining, and she was searching for a lifestyle revamp. Everything changed when she found geocaching. She began exploring her local trails, discovering caches hidden in the most unexpected places. Each successful hunt spurred her on to the next one.

Simultaneously, her newfound love for the outdoors kindled an interest in wholesome, natural food. She started carrying homemade trail mix—nuts, dried fruit, dark chocolate—on her geocaching adventures. Unbeknownst to her, she was unknowingly charting a path towards better health.

Her journey escalated when she took on the "30-Day Geocache and Green Smoothie Challenge"—hunting a geocache and concocting a green smoothie every day for a month straight. The combination of outdoor exercise and nutrient-packed power drinks transformed her life. Martha not only lost 25 pounds but also found a new passion and brought purpose back into her life.

# 11.2. Rising from the Ashes: Ed's Triumph

Ed, a software engineer, was battling work-related stress and weight gain. He yearned for a healthier lifestyle yet failed to find a fitness regimen that stuck. Then, on a camping trip, his friend introduced him to geocaching. The competitive spirit and love for problem-solving drew Ed in immediately.

Ed started geocaching every weekend, often trekking long distances to find the elusive caches. The byproduct of this adventurous pastime – not just his increasing fitness levels but also his improved mental health. In addition, Ed felt a burgeoning interest in natural nutrition as he needed more energy to walk miles into the local reserves and parks. He started researching energy-boosting yet healthy snacks.

Swapping chips and soda for whole foods like almond butter sandwiches on whole-grain bread, fruits, homemade granola bars, quinoa salads, and protein shakes allowed Ed to fuel his body in a much healthier way. The impact was tremendous - Ed managed to lose 35 pounds in six months and remarkably improve his stress levels.

# 11.3. The Adventure of Amy and Greg: A Couple's Transformation

Amy and Greg, an urban-dwelling couple, found the much-needed escape from technology and city noises when they stumbled upon geocaching. They excitedly began seeking containers in nearby parks and forests. As they started spending more time outdoors, they soon realized the need for better nutrition.

Their journey of nutritional transformation began with simple changes—swapping canned foods and fast-food meals for packed lunches with grilled chicken salads, black bean wraps, cut fruits, nuts, and plenty of water. Not only did these choices offer the much-needed energy to keep their geocaching adventures alive, but they benefited their overall health as well.

In a year of geocache-inspired fitness and nutritional changes, Amy brought her high cholesterol levels under control, and Greg lost 20 pounds and significantly increased his stamina.

# 11.4. Conclusion: Your Path Awaits

Martha, Ed, Amy, and Greg — their stories are unique, yet they resonate with each other. Incorporating geocaching into their lifestyle spurred the transformation not only on a physical level but on an emotional and mental plane as well. Their journey of fitness, bound tightly with geocaching and natural nutrition, showcases the limitless potential of this treasure-hunting activity.

Whether you are at the threshold of a healthier lifestyle or already on the path, remember that every cache you seek, each step you take, and every wholesome, natural food you opt for brings you closer to your treasure—the pinnacle of health and joy. Unearth the treasure that awaits you on the trail—around the bend, beneath the rocks, and within you. Your own success story might just be waiting for its first chapter.